CW00402643

Chair Yoga for Weight Loss

Disclaimer

Before beginning any exercise program or following the directions in this book, it is strongly recommended that you consult a physician or exercise professional.

The author and publishers of this book are not responsible for any injury or damage resulting from the use or interpretation of the information provided.

Please keep in mind that each person is unique and has different levels of physical condition and health, it is essential to listen to your body, avoid pushing yourself beyond your limits, and adapt the exercises according to your personal abilities and condition.

The proposed exercises may involve risks, and it is necessary to perform them appropriately and responsibly.

Make sure to perform the exercises in a safe and appropriate environment, using stable and suitable equipment.

Copyright © 2023 by Eden Stone

All rights reserved. No part of this publication may be reproduced, distributed, or transmitted in any form or by any means, including photocopying, recording, or other electronic or mechanical methods, without the prior written permission of the author, except in the case of brief quotations embodied in critical reviews and certain other noncommercial uses permitted by copyright law.

Mission of the Book

My mission with this book is to provide readers with the practical tools needed to take full advantage of the benefits of chair yoga as an effective means of weight loss and improved overall well-being.

I am deeply convinced that weight loss should not only be an outward goal, but also a path of inner transformation. This book was born out of my personal experience and passion for chair yoga and its potential to improve people's lives.

My intention is to offer a comprehensive and accessible guide for anyone who wishes to embrace this extraordinary approach to weight loss. I want you to discover the unique benefits of chair yoga, not only as a means to achieve a healthy weight, but also as a practice that can positively affect all aspects of your life.

Through the pages of this book, I will guide you step by step, explaining the fundamentals of chair yoga, presenting a wide range of postures, and sharing practical tips for integrating this practice into your daily life. My hope is that you will experience the joy and gratitude that accompany the attainment of a healthy body and overall well-being.

I am aware that each individual is unique, with different needs, abilities, and goals. Therefore, I strive to offer flexibility and adaptability in my proposals so that you can customize your weight-loss journey through chair yoga. You will be encouraged to explore, experiment, and find the balance that works best for you.

I sincerely hope that this book can inspire and motivate you to embrace a new vision of weight loss that goes beyond traditional patterns and focuses on the overall health of body and mind. I want you to discover the beauty of chair yoga practice and its transformative capabilities.

Get ready for a journey of discovery, growth, and change. I am here to guide and support you along the way so that you can achieve your weight-loss goals in a healthy, sustainable, and fulfilling way.

CONTENTS

INTRODUCTION

In this exploratory guide, we will dive into an extraordinary alternative approach to achieving weight loss: chair-based yoga.

Chair yoga represents a unique and highly effective method for losing weight and improving overall well-being. It differs from traditional yoga practices in that it is performed using a chair for support, making it accessible to people of all ages and physical conditions.

This innovative approach offers numerous benefits because of its adaptability to different needs and fitness levels. Whether you are a beginner or an expert, chair yoga can be customized to meet your specific needs, allowing you to progress on your weight-loss journey.

One of the most unique features of chair yoga is its ability to engage the entire body, stimulating muscles, improving flexibility, and increasing endurance. Each pose is designed to activate metabolism, promote fat burning, and tone muscles, thus helping to achieve your weight-loss goals.

In addition, chair yoga offers numerous benefits for mental and emotional health. During the practice, we focus on balancing the mind and body, which promotes stress reduction, improves concentration, and fosters an overall feeling of inner well-being.

Through this book, we will explore in detail the exercises, sequences, and approaches that will guide you on your journey to weight loss with chair yoga. You will be able to experience the benefits of this adaptive practice and discover how to integrate it into your daily life for lasting results.

Get ready to discover an innovative and accessible way to lose weight, improve your fitness, and achieve mind-body balance. Whether you are just beginning your journey or are experienced in yoga, this book will give you the practical tools you need to use chair yoga as an effective ally in your fight against excess weight.

BASIC CHAIR YOGA POSITION

Basic Concepts and Tips for Getting Started

In this chapter, we will explore the fundamentals of chair yoga, understanding the basic concepts that form the foundation of this fascinating practice. During this section, you will learn the crucial importance of proper alignment, which not only prevents injury but also maximizes the benefits of each pose.

Proper posture and alignment of the body in the chair are key elements for safe and effective practice. I will guide you in positioning your body properly, stabilizing your hands and feet, and maintaining an upright posture that promotes spinal lengthening.

In addition, we will discuss precautions to take while practicing chair yoga. Everyone has specific physical limitations and conditions, and it is essential to listen to your body and progress gradually. I will provide advice on how to interpret your body's signals and adapt the practice to your individual needs.

Chair yoga practice offers benefits beyond simple weight loss. It improves flexibility, muscle strength, and balance and promotes a sense of inner calm. This is a time devoted to taking care of oneself, both physically and mentally, and to developing greater awareness of body and mind.

A key aspect is creating a suitable space for chair yoga practice and choosing an appropriate chair—this is to ensure an enjoyable and effective practice.

Here is a detailed guide on how to prepare a suitable space for chair yoga practice and how to choose an appropriate chair:

1. Choose an ideal location: Find a quiet, well-lit area in your home where you can practice chair yoga. Make sure the space is large enough to allow you to stretch freely with your arms and legs without bumping into surrounding objects.

2. Remove obstacles: Before starting practice, move any objects or furniture that might hinder your movements. Creating an open, unobstructed space will allow you to perform the positions without restrictions.

3. Clean and freshen the area: Spend a few minutes cleaning the area where you will practice chair yoga. Remove dust and make sure the environment is fresh and pleasant. You can also add a personal touch, such as a scented candle or plant, to create a relaxing atmosphere.

4. Position the chair: Make sure you have enough space around the chair to move around comfortably. Position the chair so that it is stable and secure. Check that the four legs are resting firmly on the floor and that there is no jolting or unwanted movement.

5. Check for proper alignment: Make sure the chair is aligned correctly. The back of the chair should be straight, with the backrest supporting your spine in a neutral way. Check that the seat is at a height that allows you to keep your feet planted firmly on the floor.

6. Choose a suitable chair: Choosing the right chair is critical for an effective and safe chair yoga practice. Opt for a stable chair, preferably one without wheels, that provides you with good lumbar support. Make sure the chair is comfortable and has adequate height to allow you to maintain proper posture during the exercises.

7. Personalize your space: Add a personal touch to your practice space. You can place a blanket or pillow on the chair to make it even more comfortable. Be sure to have a water bottle and towel handy to keep you hydrated and dry during practice.

By following these simple instructions, you can create an optimal environment for chair yoga practice and ensure that you have a suitable chair that supports your body during the postures. Preparing a welcoming and functional space will allow you to fully focus on your practice and maximize the benefits of chair yoga.

FORWARD BEND

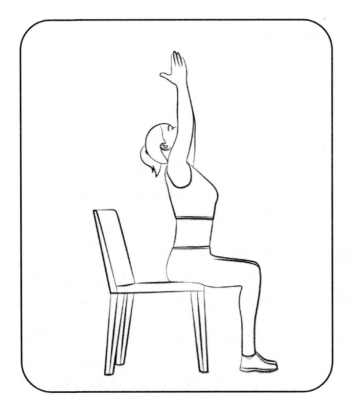 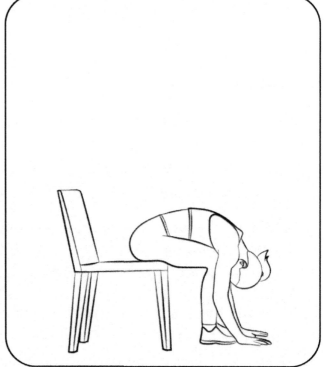

The Seated Forward Bend is a stretching exercise that primarily involves the back of the body.
It is an effective posture for relaxing the mind, stimulating digestion, and improving flexibility

Instructions for execution:

1. Sit on the edge of the chair with your back straight and legs slightly apart.
2. Make sure you have sufficient space in front of you to perform the movement.
3. Bring your arms above your head and stretch your body upward, extending your spine.
4. Exhale slowly and, keeping your back straight, start bending forward from the pelvis.
5. Proceed with the movement until you can feel a pleasant stretch in the back of your legs and lower back.
6. Hold the position for a few breaths, gradually trying to relax the muscles and deepen the stretch.
7. If possible, you can place your hands on your legs or grasp them on the sides of your feet for more stretching.

Breathing:

During the pose, focus your attention on deep, rhythmic breathing. Breathe in slowly through your nose as you extend your body upward. Gradually exhale through your nose or mouth as you bend forward, allowing the breath to guide your stretching and relaxation.

Benefits:

- Back and leg stretching: This position stretches the spine, the back muscles of the legs, and the lower back, improving flexibility and reducing muscle tension.
- Stimulation of digestion: Forward arching can promote stimulation of the digestive system and improve metabolism.
- Mental relaxation: This posture helps calm the mind, reduce stress, and promote a feeling of inner calm.
- Posture improvement: Regular performance of this exercise can help improve overall posture by reducing curvature and stiffness in the upper back.

Recommendations:

- If you have back or knee problems, change the position by reducing the range of motion.
- Listen to your body and do not force the stretch. If you feel pain or discomfort, stop or reduce the intensity of the exercise.
- Be aware of your breathing while performing the Seated Forward Bend, allowing the breath to guide the movement and relaxation.
- Practice this position on a regular basis to experience progress in flexibility and muscle relaxation over time.

CAT-COW STRETCH

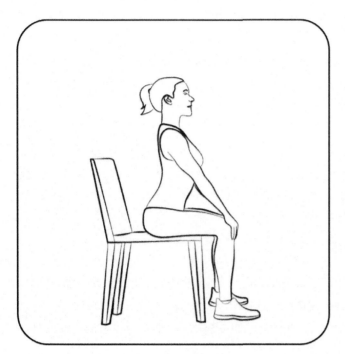
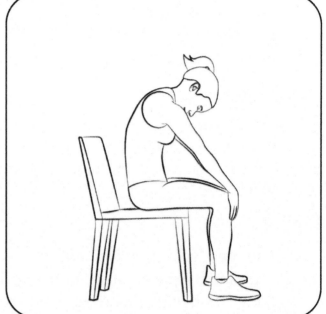

Description

The Seated Cat-Cow Stretch pose is a chair-based yoga exercise that involves a fluid sequence of movements of the spine. This pose helps relax and invigorate the back, improving flexibility and mobility of the spine.

Instructions for execution:

1. Sit on the edge of the chair, with your hands resting on your knees.

2. Make sure your back is straight and aligned.

3. Inhale deeply and lengthen the spine upward, lifting the chest slightly and pushing the shoulders back into a bowed position.

4. Hold it for a few seconds while continuing to breathe deeply.

5. Exhale slowly and rotate the pelvis forward, bringing the back into an arched position, lowering the head, and bringing the chin toward the chest.

6. Hold it for a few seconds while continuing to breathe deeply.

7. Continue alternating for a few breathing cycles, synchronizing the movements with your breathing.

Breathing:

Pay attention to conscious breathing. Inhaling, lengthen the spine and raise the chest into the "Cow" position. Exhaling, rotate the pelvis forward and lower the head into the "Cat" position. Synchronize the movement with the breathing, letting the breath guide the rhythm of the movements.

Benefits:

- Improves flexibility and mobility of the spine.

- Relaxes tension in the back and shoulders.

- Promotes strengthening of core muscles.

- Stimulates blood circulation in the back and abdomen area.

- Promotes better posture and body awareness.

Recommendations:

- Be sure to perform the Seated Cat-Cow Stretch in a smooth and controlled manner, avoiding sudden or forced movements.

- If you have back or shoulder problems, adjust the position to your individual needs and reduce the range of movement.

- Respect your limits and always listen to your body while performing.

- Practice this position regularly to improve spinal flexibility and relax the back.

SPINAL TWIST

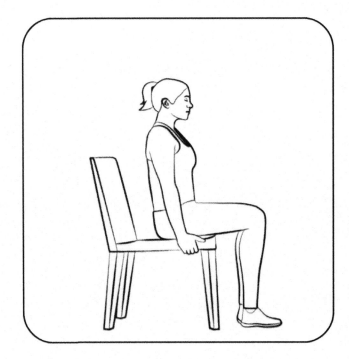
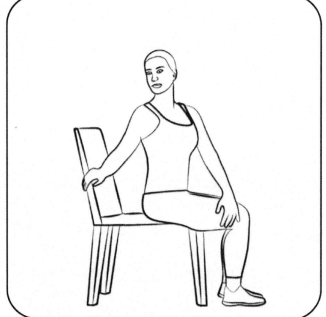

Seated Spinal Twist is a chair yoga pose that involves a rotation of the spine. This exercise helps improve spinal mobility, eases tension in the back, and aids digestion.

Instructions for execution:

1. Sit in the chair with your back straight and your feet planted firmly on the floor.

2. Bring your right hand to the armrest of the chair or the back of the chair, near the right buttock.

3. Bring your left hand to your right knee, using your arm to achieve a slight torso twist to the right.

4. Keep the spine extended and breathe deeply.

5. With each inhalation, stretch your upper body upward, and with each exhalation, perform a slight twist to the right.

6. Hold the position for 30 seconds or more, continuing to breathe deeply.

7. Slowly return to the center and repeat the movement on the other side.

Breathing:

inhale as you lengthen the spine upward and exhale as you perform the twist to the right. Try to breathe deeply and rhythmically, allowing the breath to guide the movement and promote relaxation.

Benefits:

- Improves spinal mobility and promotes paravertebral muscle lengthening.

- Reduces tension and pain in the back.

- Promotes digestion and stimulates proper functioning of internal organs.

- Promotes correct posture and body alignment.

- Promotes a feeling of relaxation and general well-being.

Recommendations:

- Be sure to keep your back straight while performing the Seated Spinal Twist.

- Avoid forcing the movement, trying instead to perform a gentle, gradual twist.

- If you experience pain or discomfort, reduce the range of motion or stop the exercise.

- Adjust the position to your individual needs, possibly using a pillow or back support if necessary.

- Be aware of your breath while performing, letting it be fluid and natural.

PIGEON POSE

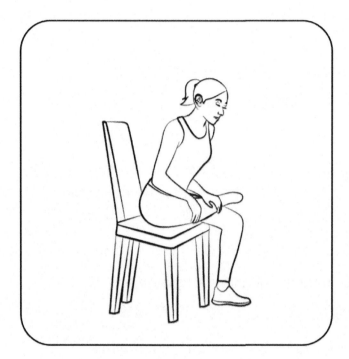 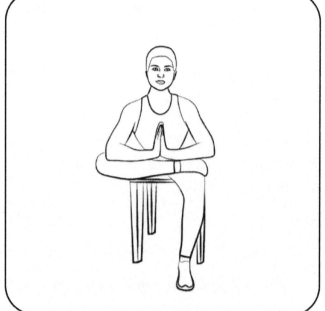

The Seated Pigeon Pose, is a chair yoga pose that focuses on stretching the muscles of the buttocks and hips. This exercise helps improve hip flexibility, reduces tension in the lower back, and relaxes the mind.

Instructions for execution:

1. Sit on the edge of the chair with your back straight and your feet planted firmly on the ground.

2. Lift your right foot and place it on your left thigh, pressing your right knee down.

3. Make sure your right foot is parallel to the side edge of the chair.

4. Keep your back straight and lengthen your spine upward.

5. If you wish to increase the intensity of the stretch, bend slightly forward from the waist, keeping your back straight.

6. Hold the position for 30 seconds or more, breathing deeply.

7. Repeat the movement on the other side, lifting the left foot and resting it on the right thigh.

Breathing:

Try to keep your breathing fluid and relaxed. As you inhale, lengthen the spine upward, and as you exhale, relax the tension in the lower back. Breathe deeply, allowing the breath to guide the movement and promote relaxation.

Benefits:

- Stretches and relaxes the muscles of the buttocks and hips.

- Improves hip flexibility and lower back mobility.

- Reduces tension in the lower back.

- Promotes correct posture and alignment of the body.

- Promotes a feeling of relaxation and calm.

Recommendations:

- Be sure to keep your back straight while performing.

- Do not force the movement, respecting your body's limits and maintaining a comfortable stretch.

- If you experience pain or discomfort, reduce the range of motion or stop the exercise.

- Possibly use a pillow or support under the raised buttock to improve comfort and alignment.

- Be aware of your breath while performing, letting it be fluid and natural.

EAGLE POSE

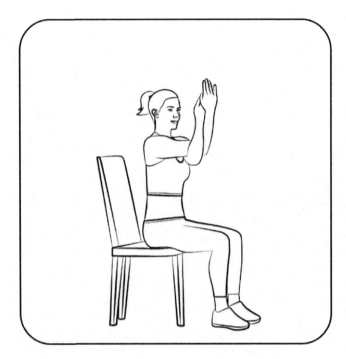

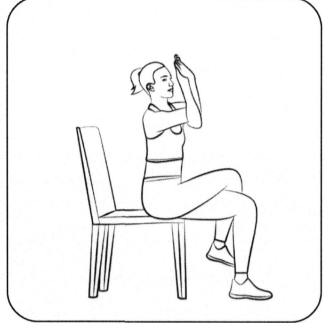

Description

The Seated Eagle Pose is a chair yoga pose that involves a twisting of the torso and twisting of the arms to promote relaxation and strengthening of the body.

Instructions for execution:

1. Sit on the edge of the chair with your back straight and your feet resting firmly on the floor.

2. Bring your arms in front of you, parallel to the floor, palms facing each other.

3. Cross your right arm over your left arm, bringing your elbows to touch and your palms to touch each other. You can also wrap your right wrist around your left wrist for an intensification of the position.

4. Cross your right leg over your left leg, bringing your right foot behind your left calf.

5. Bring the shoulders down and move the shoulder blades away from the neck to open the chest.

6. Hold the position for 5-10 deep breaths, feeling a slight twist in the upper body.

7. Release the position and repeat on the opposite side, crossing the left arm over the right arm.

Breathing:

Breathe regularly and deeply. Inhale as you prepare for the pose and then exhale as you enter the twist. Keep breathing smoothly throughout the execution, allowing the breath to guide the movement and expansion of the body.

Benefits:

- Stabilizes and lengthens the spine.

- Promotes mobility of the shoulders and arms.

- Stimulates blood and lymphatic circulation in the upper body.

- Promotes relaxation and stress reduction.

Recommendations:

- If you have problems with your shoulders or arms, adapt the position to your needs or ask a yoga instructor for advice.

- Always listen to your body and work within your comfortable range of motion.

- Avoid forcing the twist and remember to maintain smooth breathing throughout the practice.

Note: The Seated Eagle Pose is an advanced chair yoga pose that requires good shoulder and arm mobility.

LEG RAISE

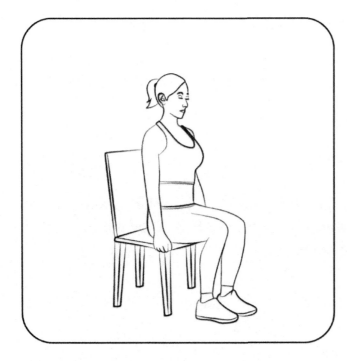 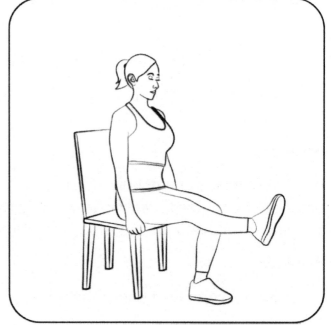

Description

The Seated Leg Raise is a chair yoga pose that aims to strengthen leg muscles, improve stability, and stimulate blood circulation in the legs.

Instructions for execution:

1. Sit in the chair with your back straight and legs bent at a right angle, feet planted firmly on the floor.

2. Rest your hands on the sides of the chair to maintain balance.

3. Inhaling, slowly lift one leg so that the foot is off the floor. Keep the leg straight without locking the knee.

4. Hold the position for a few seconds, feeling the work of the raised leg muscles.

5. Exhaling, gently lower the leg to a sitting position.

6. Repeat the leg lift with the other leg.

Breathing:

During the Seated Leg Raise, breathe naturally. You can inhale as you raise your leg and exhale as you lower it. Keep your breathing regular and effortless.

Benefits:

- Strengthens leg muscles, particularly the quadriceps and adductors.

- Promotes improved balance and stability.

- Stimulates blood circulation in the legs.

- Helps tone the legs and improve the overall strength of the lower limbs.

Recommendations:

- Be sure to keep your back straight while performing.

- Start with light leg lifts and gradually increase the intensity depending on your ability and fitness level.

- If you experience pain or overexertion, stop the exercise and adjust the position to your needs.

EXTENDED TRIANGLE POSE

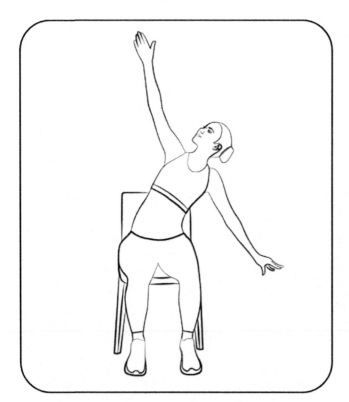 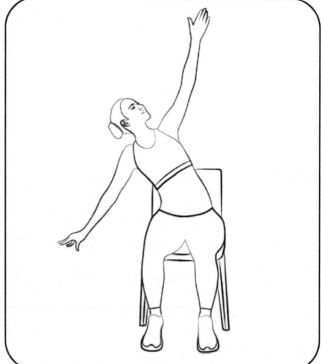

Description

The Extended Triangle Pose is a position that works on lateral flexibility of the spine while also stimulating the muscles of the legs and abdomen. This pose helps stretch the hips and improve body balance.

Instructions for execution:

1. Sit in the chair with your back straight and your feet resting on the floor.

2. Bring legs into a slightly spread position, with feet parallel to each other.

3. Raise your right arm upward, stretching it toward the ceiling.

4. Exhale slowly and tilt the torso to the left, bringing the right arm above the head, while the left hand extends toward the floor.

5. Hold the position for 3–5 deep breaths, trying to keep your back straight and torso extended.

6. Inhale slowly and return to the center.

7. Repeat the movement on the opposite side, lifting the left arm upward and tilting the torso to the right.

Breathing:

Try to maintain smooth, controlled breathing. Inhaling, extend your arm upward and feel the lateral stretch of your body. Exhaling, deepen the position and relax the body.

Benefits:

- Stretches the lateral muscles of the torso and spine.

- Promotes open hips and improved balance.

- Stimulates blood circulation in the trunk region.

- Promotes flexibility of the spine.

- Helps to relax the mind and reduce stress.

Recommendations:

- If you have back or shoulder problems, change the position by keeping your torso slightly more upright.

- Avoid forcing lateral tilt if you experience pain or discomfort.

- You can adjust the intensity of the lateral stretch by tilting your torso more or less.

- Maintain proper spinal alignment, avoiding excessive arching of the back.

FISH POSE

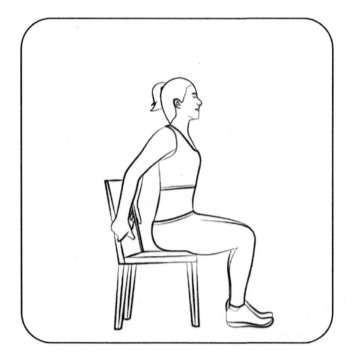 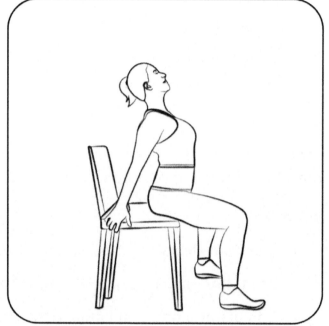

This pose is a variation of the traditional Fish Pose (Matsyasana) adapted for chair yoga practice. Seated Fish Pose offers numerous benefits for the body and mind, including opening the chest and shoulders, strengthening the spine, and relaxing the body.

Instructions for execution:

1. Sit on the edge of the chair with your back straight and your feet planted firmly on the ground.

2. Bring your hands to your thighs and align your spine.

3. Bring the shoulders back and down, stretching the neck upward to create a slight curve in the lower back.

4. Bring your hands to the chair behind you, palms facing down.

5. Press your hands into the chair and lift your chest upward, opening your chest and shoulders.

6. Relax your neck and head, keeping your gaze upward or toward the ceiling.

7. Breathe deeply and feel the opening of your chest and shoulders as you hold the position for 5–10 breaths.

8. To exit the position, slowly release the pressure of your hands on the chair, returning your body to the upright position.

Breathing:

Conscious breathing during Seated Fish Pose consists of taking slow, deep breaths, trying to lengthen the inhalation and exhalation. This breathing helps to relax the body and focus the mind during practice.

Benefits:

- Opening the chest and shoulders: The position helps stretch and open the chest and shoulder muscles, improving posture and relieving accumulated tension.

- Strengthening the spine: The curve created in the lower back during the position helps strengthen and lengthen the spine.

- Relaxation of body and mind, relieving stress and mental fatigue.

- Stimulation of the respiratory system, allowing the lungs to fully expand.

Recommendations:

- If you have back or neck problems, be sure not to force the curve in your lower back too hard.
- Modify the position according to your individual needs and limitations.
- Always listen to your body and work within your comfortable range of motion.

LOTUS POSE

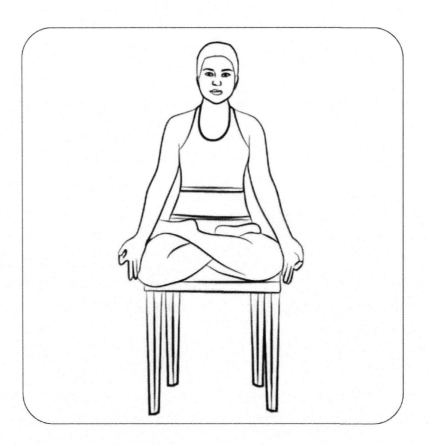

Description

The Seated Lotus Pose is a variation of the classic "Lotus Pose" in yoga. This pose involves a stretch of the legs and requires flexibility of the hips and knees.

Instructions for execution:

1. Sit on the edge of the chair with your back straight and your legs stretched out in front of you.
2. Bend the right knee and bring the right foot to the left thigh, as close to the groin as possible.
3. Repeat the same movement with the left knee, bringing the left foot onto the right thigh, as close to the groin as possible.
4. Make sure both knees are in contact with the chair and the soles of the feet are pointing upward.
5. Rest your hands on your thighs or join your hands in a mudra (symbolic hand gesture) of your choice.
6. Keep your spine straight, chin slightly retracted and eyes closed or fixed on a fixed point.
7. Relax the muscles of the face, shoulders, and pelvis.
8. Breathe deeply and hold the position for a few breaths, gradually trying to relax the legs and hips.

Breathing:

Maintain deep, regular breathing. Inhaling, lengthen the spine upward. Exhaling, relax the body and deepen the position.

Benefits:

- Stimulates flexibility in the hips, knees, and legs.
- Promotes correct posture and lengthens the spine.
- Calms the mind and promotes concentration.
- Helps relax the body and reduce stress.

Recommendations:

- If you have difficulty performing the full pose, you can start with a more accessible variation, such as the Half Lotus Pose, keeping only one leg crossed over the other.
- Listen to your body and do not force the position. Respect your limits and proceed gradually.
- The Seated Lotus Pose takes time and practice to perform correctly. Be patient with yourself and accept your current level of flexibility.
- You can use pillows or supports under the knees or buttocks to make the position more comfortable, if necessary.
- If you have difficulty maintaining balance or experience pain while performing, stop the position and try again later.

STRENGTH EXERCISES

CHAIR SQUATS

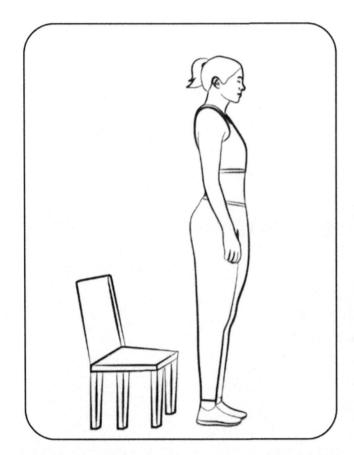 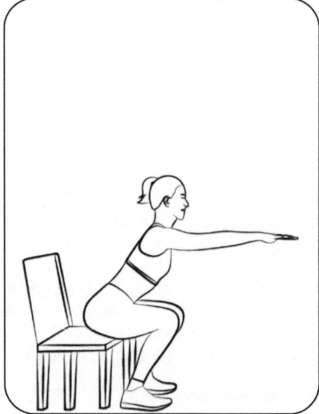

Description

Chair Squats are an effective exercise to strengthen leg and gluteal muscles using a chair as a reference point. This functional movement helps improve leg strength, core stability, and hip mobility.

Instructions for execution:

1. Place a stable chair behind you, keeping your feet shoulder-width apart.

2. Fix your gaze straight ahead, align your back, and keep your abs contracted for good posture.

3. Start by slowly bending your knees and lowering yourself toward the chair, as if you were going to sit down.

4. Keep your heels resting on the ground and distribute your weight evenly on both feet.

5. Continue bending until your buttocks barely touch the chair, keeping tension on your leg muscles.

6. Pause for a second in the lowest position, then push through the heels to slowly return to standing, extending the legs.

7. Repeat the movement for the desired number of repetitions.

Breathing:

Inhale as you descend, maintaining controlled breathing. Exhale as you push through your heels to return to standing.

Benefits:

- Strengthens leg muscles, including the quadriceps, hamstrings, and glutes.

- Helps improve core balance and stability.

- Promotes increased functional strength for daily activities such as walking, climbing stairs, and getting out of a chair.

- Helps improve hip mobility and leg flexibility.

Recommendations:

- Make sure the chair is stable and not slippery before performing Chair Squats.

- Adapt the depth of movement to your ability and comfort. Start with a range of motion that you are comfortable with and, over time, try to gradually increase the depth.

- Always maintain good posture during the exercise, avoiding bending your back forward or leaning your knees forward beyond your toes.

INCLINED PUSH-UP

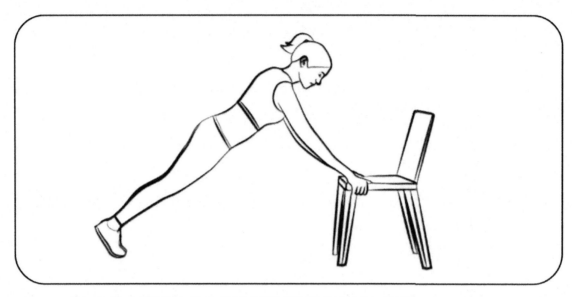

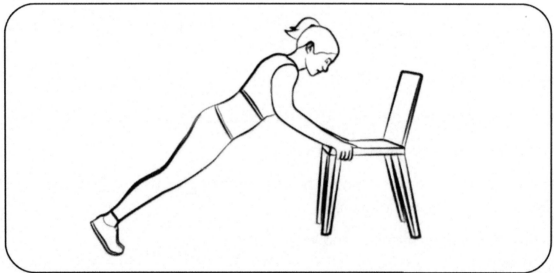

Description

Inclined Chair Push-ups are an exercise that aims to strengthen the muscles of the chest, shoulders, and arms. Using a chair for support, this variation of traditional push-ups offers an adapted and accessible option for training the upper body.

Instructions for execution:

1. Place a stable chair in front of you, with the back of the chair facing away from you and with at least a few feet of space behind you.

2. Rest your hands on the edges of the chair, slightly wider than shoulder width apart, with fingers pointing forward.

3. Extend your legs behind you, keeping your body in a straight line and supporting your weight on your toes.

4. Flex your elbows and lower your chest toward the chair, keeping your body in alignment. Try to bring your chest as close to the chair as possible without touching it.

5. Pause for a moment in the lowest position, then push through your hands to return to the starting position, fully extending your arms.

6. Repeat the movement for the desired number of repetitions.

Breathing:

Inhale as you lower your chest toward the chair and exhale as you push through your hands to return to the starting position.

Benefits:

- Strengthens the muscles of the chest, shoulders, and arms, including the deltoids, pectorals, and triceps.

- Helps improve core stability and balance.

- Promotes the development of functional strength in the upper body.

Recommendations:

- Make sure the chair is stable and firm before performing Inclined Chair Push-ups.

- Start with a prone position that allows you to maintain good form during the exercise. Gradually increase the incline as you feel stronger.

- Keep the body in a straight line while performing, avoiding dropping the hips or raising the butt high.

- Adapt the exercise if needed to suit your fitness level.

CHAIRPLANK

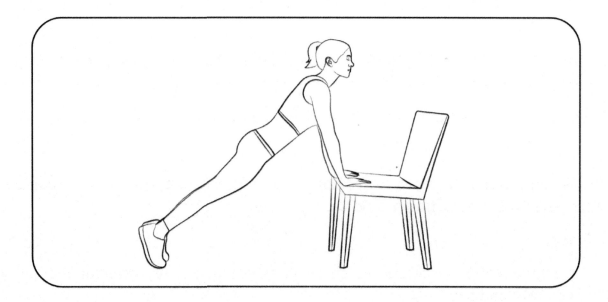

Description

The Plank on the Chair is an effective exercise for strengthening core muscles, including the abdominals, back muscles, and shoulder stabilizers. Using a chair for support, this variation of the traditional plank offers an adapted and accessible way to train body stability and strength.

Instructions for execution:

1. Place a stable chair in front of you.

2. Rest your forearms on the chair, with your elbows under your shoulders and your hands slightly clasped.

3. Extend your legs behind you, keeping your body in a straight line and supporting your weight on your feet or knees.

4. Contract your core and buttock muscles to keep your body stable and aligned.

5. Hold the plank position for as long as desired, trying to maintain good form and regular breathing.

6. Relax the body slowly and rest for a moment before repeating the exercise.

Breathing:

Breathe in a controlled and regular manner during the plank. Try to maintain deep, steady breathing to support muscle stability and control.

Benefits:

- Strengthens core muscles, including abdominals, back muscles, and shoulder stabilizers.

- Improves trunk stability and posture.

- Promotes the development of functional strength and balance.

Recommendations:

- Make sure the chair is stable and firm before performing the Plank on the Chair.

- Start with a position that allows you to maintain good form during the exercise. Gradually increase the duration of the plank as you feel stronger.

- Keep the body in a straight line while performing, avoiding dropping the hips or raising the butt high.

- Adapt the exercise if needed to suit your fitness level.

CHAIR TRICEPS

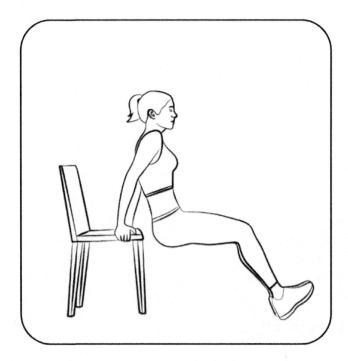 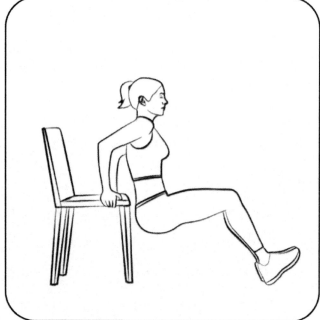

Description

Chair Triceps are a great way to strengthen and tone the back muscles of the arms. Using a chair for support, these exercises allow you to focus on working your triceps specifically in a safe and effective way.

Instructions for execution:

1. Place a stable chair behind you.

2. Sit in the chair and place your hands on the edge of the chair next to your hips, fingers pointing downward.

3. Move your body away from the chair by lifting your buttocks and moving your feet forward until your legs are straight and your heels rest on the floor.

4. Flex your elbows and lower your body toward the floor, bending your elbows. Keep the elbows close to the body.

5. When your elbows form an angle of about 90 degrees, push hard on your hands to extend your elbows and return to the starting position.

6. Repeat the movement for the desired number of repetitions.

Breathing:

Exhale as you lift your body and contract your triceps and inhale as you return to the starting position. Maintain controlled and regular breathing while performing the exercise.

Benefits:

*   Strengthens and tones the triceps muscles, contributing to more toned and defined arms.

*   Improves functional strength of the upper limbs.

*   Promotes the development of balance and trunk stability.

Recommendations:

*   Make sure the chair is stable and firm before performing triceps exercises in the chair.

*   Start with a range of motion that allows you to maintain good form and avoid excessive tension on the elbows and shoulders.

*   Maintain an upright posture while performing, avoiding arching your back or pushing forward with your shoulders.

CHAIR STEP-UP

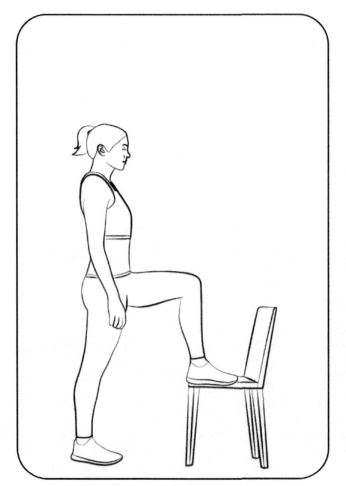 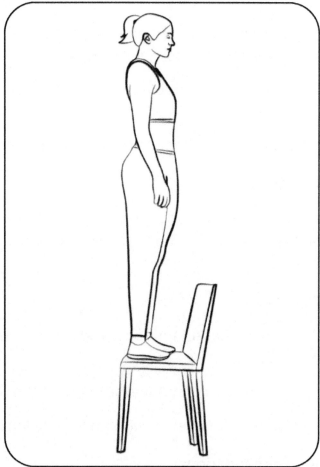

Description

Chair Step-ups are an effective exercise for training the lower body, particularly the leg and gluteal muscles. Using the chair as a reference point, this exercise helps improve strength, stability, and coordination.

Instructions for execution:

1. Place a stable chair in front of you.

2. Rest the right foot entirely on the surface of the chair, keeping the heel firmly anchored.

3. Push through the heel of the right foot and lift the body upward, bringing the left foot to the chair.

4. Be sure to keep your weight on the heel of the foot that is on the chair and control the movement.

5. Pause in the position where both feet are on the chair, then slowly come down, bringing the left foot back to the floor.

6. Repeat the movement, alternating feet throughout the entire set.

Breathing:

Perform controlled breathing during the exercise. Exhale as you push through the heel to rise in the chair and inhale as you descend.

Benefits:

- Strengthens leg muscles, particularly the quadriceps, hamstrings, and gluteal muscles.

- Improves stability, balance, and coordination.

- Promotes metabolism and may contribute to weight loss.

- It can be adapted to different fitness levels by varying the height of the chair or the use of additional weights.

Recommendations:

- Make sure the chair is stable and firm.

- Keep your back straight while performing the exercise and control the movement.

- Start with a chair of appropriate height for your fitness level and gradually increase the difficulty by stretching the supporting leg or using additional weights.

- Avoid pushing through the toe. Instead, focus on the heel to lift you up in the chair.

- Adapt the exercise for your fitness level if needed by varying the height of the chair or adding weights.

REVERSE PLANK

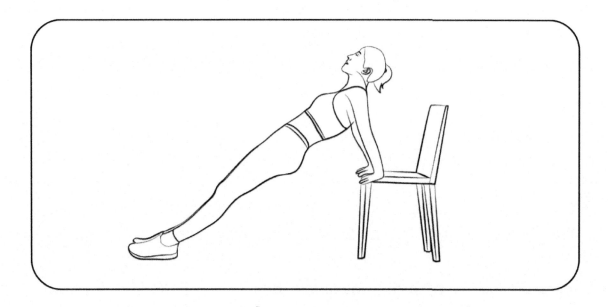

Description

The Chair Reverse Plank is an exercise that primarily involves the upper body, including the muscles of the arms, shoulders, and core. Using the chair as support, this exercise helps improve strength, stability, and flexibility.

Instructions for execution:

1. Place the chair behind you and sit on the edge of the chair with your legs stretched out in front of you.

2. Rest your hands on the edge of the chair, fingers pointing toward your body.

3. Lift your buttocks off the chair, keeping your arms extended and legs outstretched.

4. Keeping a straight line from chest to knees, contract core muscles to stabilize the body.

5. Be sure to keep your shoulders relaxed and lowered, avoiding raising them toward your ears.

6. Hold the position for a few seconds, breathing in a controlled manner.

7. Slowly release the position by lowering the buttocks onto the chair.

Breathing:

Perform controlled breathing during the exercise. Inhale as you lift your buttocks out of the chair and exhale as you return to the starting position.

Benefits:

- Strengthens the muscles of the arms, shoulders, and core.

- Improves trunk stability and shoulder flexibility.

- Promotes good posture and stretches the front muscles of the body.

- Stimulates the nervous system and can help improve body awareness.

Recommendations:

- Make sure the chair is stable and strong before performing the reverse plank.

- Maintain good form during the exercise, avoiding dropping your head back or excessively arching your lower back.

- If you have problems with your shoulders or wrists, you can modify the exercise by bending your elbows slightly or using a hand support, such as a yoga block.

- Start with a short holding time and gradually increase the duration as you develop strength and endurance.

LEG PUSH-UP

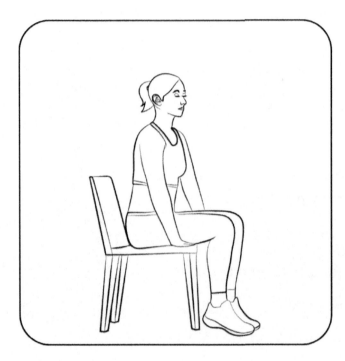 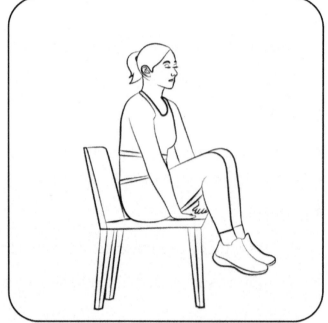

Chair Leg Push-ups are an effective exercise for working the leg muscles, particularly the lower abdominals and hip flexor muscles. This position, performed while sitting in a chair, helps improve leg strength and flexibility, contributing to muscle tone and overall well-being.

Instructions for execution:

1. Sit in a stable chair with both feet resting firmly on the floor.

2. Be sure to maintain good posture, with a straight back and relaxed shoulders.

3. Bring your hands to the sides of the chair to get good support and maintain balance.

4. Lift both feet off the floor, bending the knees toward the chest.

5. Hold the position for a few seconds.

6. Slowly, extend your legs downward, repositioning your feet on the floor.

7. Repeat the movement for the desired number of repetitions.

Breathing:

While performing the Chair Leg Push-ups, breathe in a controlled and natural way. Inhale as you lift your legs toward your chest and exhale as you extend your legs downward.

Benefits:

- Strengthens the lower abdominals and hip flexor muscles.

- Improves leg flexibility and range of motion of the hip joint.

- Contributes to muscle tone and leg definition.

- Helps improve balance and core stability.

- It can be adapted to different physical abilities by adjusting the number of repetitions and duration of the position.

Recommendations:

- Use a stable, sturdy chair to perform this exercise safely.

- Start with a comfortable range of motion, bending your knees toward your chest to the extent you feel comfortable.

- Maintain good posture while performing, keeping your back straight and shoulders relaxed.

- Adapt the exercise to your physical abilities if needed by adjusting the number of repetitions and duration of the position.

CALF RAISES

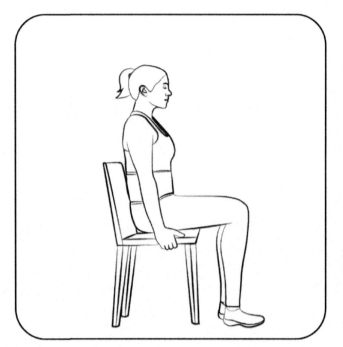
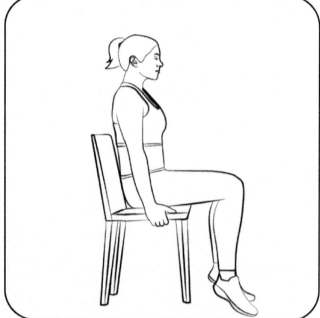

Description

Chair Calf Raises are a targeted exercise to strengthen the calf muscles, helping to improve lower extremity stability and promoting better leg strength and definition. This position, performed using a chair as a support point, provides an effective way to work the calf muscles without the use of specific equipment. It is a convenient exercise to perform anywhere you have access to a stable chair

Instructions for execution:

1. Place a stable chair in front of you, at a distance that allows you to rest your hands comfortably on its surface.

2. Stand with your legs slightly apart and your feet in line with your shoulders.

3. Rest your hands on the front edge of the chair to maintain balance and stability during the exercise.

4. Slowly lift your heels off the floor, pushing upward with your calf muscles.

5. Keep the contraction of the calf muscles at the top of the movement for a few seconds.

6. Slowly lower your heels to the floor, returning to the starting position.

7. Repeat the movement for the desired number of repetitions.

Breathing:

While performing calf raises in the chair, breathe in a controlled manner. Inhale as you raise your heels and exhale as you lower them toward the floor.

Benefits:

- Strengthens the calf muscles, including the gastrocnemius muscle and soleus muscle.

- Improves lower limb stability and muscle coordination.

- Helps develop endurance and tone in the legs.

Recommendations:

- Use a firm, stable chair to perform the exercise correctly.

- Maintain an upright posture while performing, with a straight back and relaxed shoulders.

- Focus on contracting the calf muscles during the lifting action.

- Start with a comfortable range of motion and gradually increase.

- Adapt this exercise to your physical abilities if needed by adjusting the number of repetitions and intensity of the exercise.

ARM EXTENSIONS

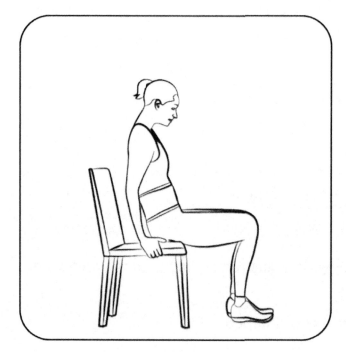 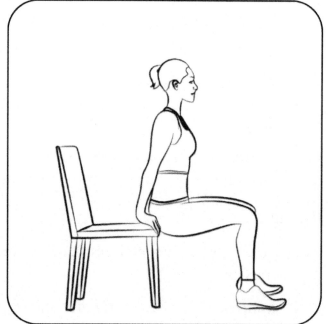

Chair Arm Extensions are a simple but effective exercise to strengthen arm muscles and improve shoulder stability. This exercise is performed using a chair as a support to lift the body and work the upper limbs.

Instructions for execution:

1. Sit in the chair with your back straight and legs bent at a right angle, feet resting firmly on the floor.

2. Place your hands on the edges of the chair, with fingers pointing downward and palms resting on the surface of the chair.

3. Push down with your hands and lift your body off the chair, keeping your arms slightly bent.

4. Fully extend your arms, keeping your elbows close to your body. Shoulders should be relaxed and lowered.

5. Hold this position for a few seconds, trying to stabilize the body and maintain proper alignment.

6. Then slowly lower your body back to the starting position, bending your elbows slightly.

Breathing:

While performing the Chair Arm Extensions, inhale as you raise your body and hold your breath while holding the position. Exhale as you lower your body toward the chair.

Benefits:

- Strengthens arm muscles, including triceps, biceps, and deltoids.

- Improves shoulder stability and core strength.

- Promotes correct posture and body alignment.

- Helps develop the overall strength of the upper limbs.

Recommendations:

- Start with a number of repetitions appropriate for your strength level and gradually increase the intensity.

- Always maintain the correct posture, avoiding bending forward or rounding your shoulders.

- Be careful not to lift your body too high and avoid straining your neck or shoulder muscles.

CARDIO EXERCISES

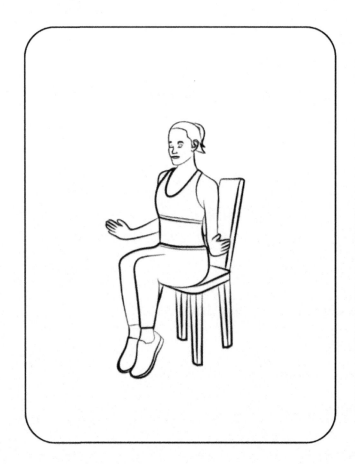
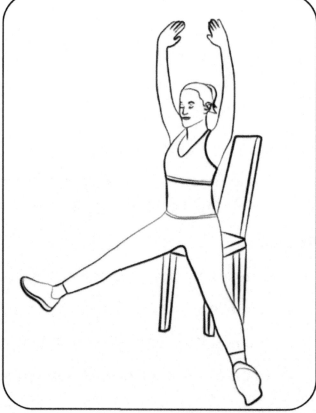

Description

The Jumping Jacks Session is a variation of traditional exercise adapted to be performed in the chair. It involves the entire body, providing an effective cardiovascular workout and helping to burn calories.

Instructions for execution:

1. Sit in the chair with your back straight and your feet resting on the floor.

2. Place your hands on your thighs or keep them slightly raised on your hips.

3. In a fluid motion, simultaneously open your legs outward and raise your arms above your head.

4. Return to starting position, lowering arms and bringing legs together.

5. Repeat the movement continuously for the desired duration of the exercise.

Breathing:

Inhale during the starting position and exhale when you open your legs and raise your arms. Maintain regular, controlled breathing during the exercise.

Benefits:

- Stimulates blood circulation and metabolism.

- Improves cardiovascular and pulmonary endurance.

- Involves several muscle groups, including the legs, abdominals, arms, and shoulders.

- Promotes improved balance and coordination.

Recommendations:

- Maintain correct posture with a straight back and slightly contracted abs.

- Adapt the range of motion to your personal ability and comfort.

- Remember to perform the exercise in a safe and controlled manner, adapting it to your fitness level and individual abilities.

HIGH KNEES

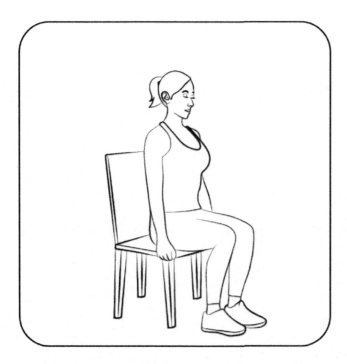 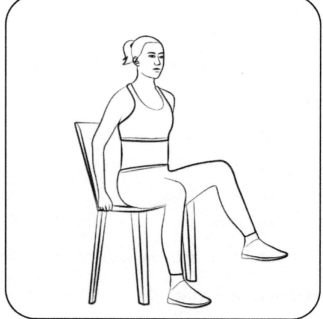

Sitting High Knees are a cardiovascular exercise that involves the action of alternately raising the knees in a seated position in the chair. This dynamic movement helps to increase heart rate and stimulate metabolism.

Instructions for execution:

1. Sit in the chair with your back straight and your feet resting on the floor.

2. Keep your hands on your hips or position them slightly raised on your thighs.

3. Lift one leg at a time, bending the knee and bringing the knee to the chest.

4. Lower one leg and raise the other leg, alternating the movement of the knees quickly and continuously.

5. Continue performing the movement, trying to maintain a steady rhythm.

Breathing:

Maintain regular breathing during the exercise, trying to breathe in a controlled manner. You can inhale and exhale synchronously with the movement of your knees.

Benefits:

- Increases heart rate and stimulates blood circulation.

- Improves cardiovascular endurance and lung capacity.

- Involves the muscles of the lower limbs, including the quadriceps, adductors, and calves.

- Helps strengthen abdominal muscles and improve core stability.

Recommendations:

- Maintain an upright and stable posture in the chair during exercise.

- Try to lift your knees as high as possible, bringing them toward your chest.

- Adapt the intensity of the exercise to your individual ability by gradually increasing the pace or knee height.

- If you have difficulty maintaining a fast pace, you can perform the knee movement more slowly, focusing on contracting the muscles involved.

Note: Experiment with different variations, such as lifting the knees diagonally or bringing them to the sides, to increase the challenge and engage different muscle groups.

JUMP SQUAT

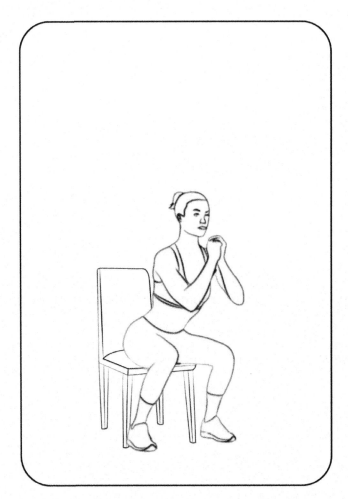 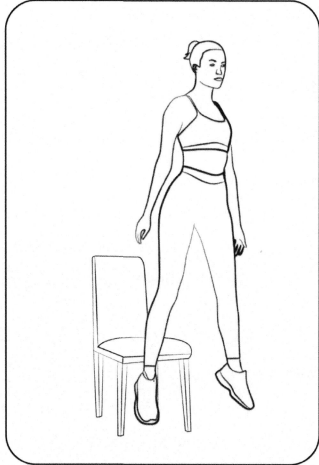

Description

Sitting Jump Squats are a cardiovascular exercise involving a combination of squats and jumps, performed in the seated position in a chair. This dynamic movement helps to increase heart rate, stimulate metabolism, and strengthen lower limb muscles.

Instructions for execution:

1. Sit in the chair with your back straight and your feet resting on the floor.

2. Bring your hands to your thighs or cross your arms over your chest to keep your balance.

3. Lift your buttocks slightly off the chair, keeping your feet on the floor.

4. Bend your knees and lower your pelvis in a squat motion, as if you were about to get up from your chair.

5. In an explosive movement, forcefully push yourself upward, lifting your feet off the ground and making a vertical leap.

6. Land softly by returning to the squat position in the chair.

7. Repeat the movement smoothly and continuously, performing jump squats in succession.

Breathing: Maintain regular breathing during the exercise. You can inhale as you lower into the squat position and exhale as you perform the jump.

Benefits:

- Increases heart rate and stimulates blood circulation.

- Improves cardiovascular endurance and lung capacity.

- Strengthens the muscles of the legs, including the quadriceps and buttocks.

- Helps strengthen the abdominals and core muscles.

Recommendations:

- Make sure you have a stable, sturdy chair on which to perform the exercise.

- Maintain good posture during the exercise, keeping your back straight and torso elevated.

- Start with controlled movements, without jumping, to get the body used to the squat position in the chair.

- Progressively, increase the intensity, pushing the body upward with force and precision.

- If you have knee or joint problems, consult your doctor before performing Sitting Jump Squats.

- The Sitting Jump Squats are an advanced exercise that requires strength and coordination.

BOXER PUNCHES

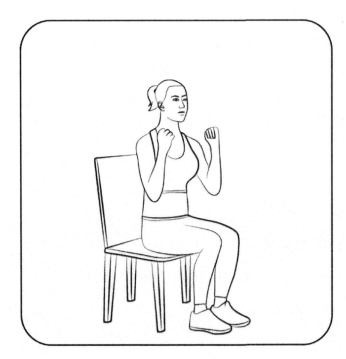 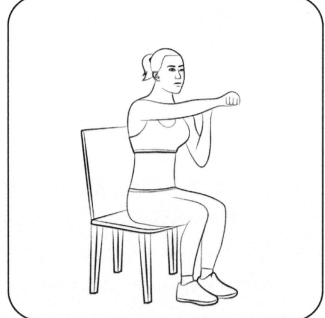

Description

The Seated Boxer Punches are a cardiovascular exercise that simulates the movements of boxers during a workout. This exercise, performed in the seated position in the chair, involves the use of the upper limbs and helps improve cardiovascular endurance, coordination, and strength of the arm and shoulder muscles.

Instructions for execution:

1. Sit in the chair with your back straight, your feet resting on the floor, and your hands relaxed at your sides.

2. Raise both arms by bending the elbows and bringing the fists close to the face.

3. Maintain a light closed fist with fingers and knuckles aligned.

4. Begin the movement by pushing the right arm forward, fully extending the arm and rotating the fist to point it outward.

5. Pull your right arm back toward your face while simultaneously pushing your left arm forward, following the same movement.

6. Continue alternating the punches of the two arms in a fast, rhythmic motion.

Breathing:

Breathe naturally during the exercise, trying to maintain a regular rhythm. You can exhale slightly during the punch to express strength.

Benefits:

- Increases heart rate and improves cardiovascular endurance.
- Tones and strengthens the muscles of the arms, shoulders, and chest.
- Helps improve coordination and agility.
- Promotes stress release and increased energy.

Recommendations:

- Make sure you have a stable chair and position yourself securely before starting the exercise.
- Start with controlled movements to get the body used to the movement.
- Focus on performing the movement correctly, making sure to keep your elbows bent and shoulders relaxed.
- You can adjust the intensity of the exercise by increasing or decreasing the speed of the punches.

CROSS PUNCHES

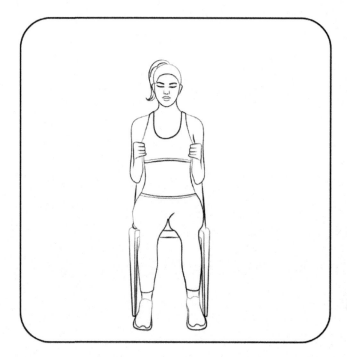 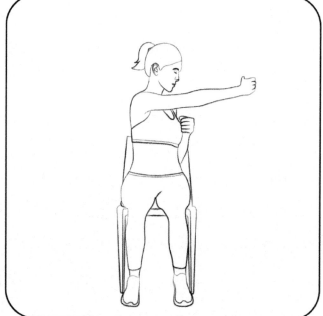

Seated Cross Punches are an exercise that involves the upper trunk and upper limbs, providing an excellent upper body workout. This exercise is based on performing cross punches, which work the upper limbs and activate the core muscles.

Instructions for execution:

1. Sit in the chair in an upright position, with your feet resting firmly on the floor.

2. Keep your arms flexed, with your fists close to your chest and your hands at shoulder level.

3. Begin the movement by extending the right arm toward the left side of the body, simulating a cross-fist.

4. Return to the center and then extend the left arm toward the right side of the body, making another cross-fist.

5. Continue alternating cross-fists from side to side, keeping a brisk pace and good form.

Breathing:

Exhale while extending the arm and inhale during the return to the starting position. Maintain regular, controlled breathing throughout the exercise.

Benefits:

- Strengthens upper limbs, including shoulder muscles, biceps, and triceps.

- Involves core muscles to maintain a stable posture while performing.

- Increases muscular and cardiovascular endurance.

- Improves coordination and agility.

- Burns calories and promotes weight loss.

Recommendations:

- Maintain an upright posture, with a straight back and slightly contracted abs.

- Be sure to perform the movement with control and without excessive muscle tension.

- You can adjust the intensity of the exercise by increasing or decreasing the speed of the punches or increasing the duration of the exercise.

- Focus on proper execution of the movement, making sure your punches are powerful and controlled.

MOUNTAIN CLIMBERS

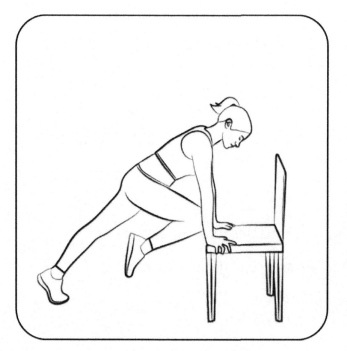 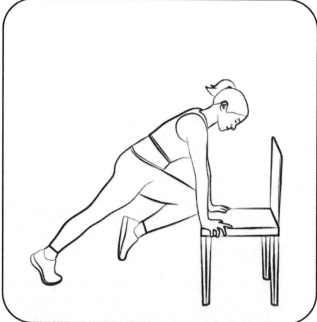

Description

The Chair Mountain Climbers are a dynamic exercise that involves several body parts, including the abs, arms, and legs. In this position, the hands are placed on the chair, creating a prone plank position. The bending movements of the knees simulate running in place, creating an effective cardiovascular workout.

Instructions for execution:

1. Place your hands on the chair, slightly wider than shoulder width apart, keeping your arms extended.

2. Align your body in a prone plank position, with your legs extended behind you and your weight evenly distributed on your hands and feet.

3. Bring one knee toward the chest, bending the leg and bringing the foot as close to the hands as possible.

4. Extend the bent leg backward, restoring the prone plank position.

5. At the same time, bring the other knee toward the chest, performing a running motion in place with the legs.

6. Continue to alternate leg movements quickly, keeping a steady, controlled pace.

Breathing: You can exhale as you bring your knee toward your chest and inhale as you extend your leg backward.

Benefits:

- Works the abdominals, strengthening the core and promoting trunk stability.

- Involves the arms and shoulders, helping to develop upper body strength.

- Develops cardiovascular endurance and promotes caloric expenditure.

- Improves coordination and balance.

- It can be adapted to different physical abilities by adjusting the speed and intensity of the exercise.

Recommendations:

- Make sure the chair is stable and securely positioned before performing the exercise.

- Maintain correct posture throughout the movement, with your back straight and abs slightly contracted.

- Start with a moderate pace and gradually increase the intensity and speed, depending on your personal ability.

- Be careful to maintain control of the movement and not to perform it too quickly or with sudden movements.

- Adapt this exercise to your physical abilities by adjusting its speed and intensity.

RUSSIAN TWIST

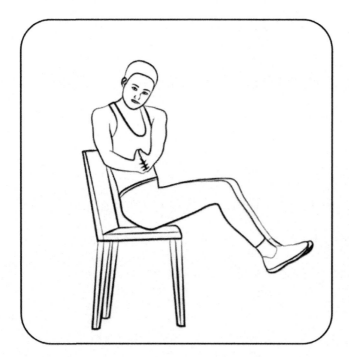 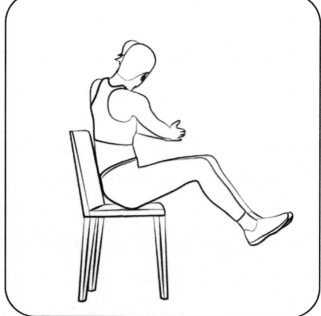

The Russian Twist in the Chair is an exercise that aims to strengthen the oblique abdominals and improve trunk stability.

Instructions for execution:

1. Sit on the edge of the chair, with your back straight, knees bent, and feet lifted off the floor.

2. Hold your hands in front of your chest, with your elbows slightly bent.

3. Begin the movement by rotating the torso to the right, bringing the hands toward the right side of the body.

4. Slow down the movement and return to center, then rotate the torso to the left, bringing the hands toward the left side of the body.

5. Continue alternating rotations from side to side, maintaining a smooth and controlled rhythm.

Breathing:

Exhale as you rotate your torso to one side and inhale as you return to the center, preparing for the next rotation.

Benefits:

- Strengthens oblique abdominals, helping to define the waist and improve trunk stability.

- Improves mobility of the spine and flexibility of the torso.

- Engages back muscles, promoting correct posture and preventing back pain.

- Develops coordination and balance.

Recommendations:

- Maintain an upright posture throughout the exercise, with a straight back and slightly contracted abs.

- Start with slow, controlled movements, focusing on correct execution of the movement.

- To increase the intensity, you can hold a weight or object in your hands during the movement.

- Avoid sudden or unbalanced movements, always maintaining control of the movement.

HOLISTIC APPROACH TO WEIGHT LOSS

Important Background Information

The goal of this chapter is to provide a holistic view on weight loss, encompassing not only the physical, but also the mental and emotional aspects that can influence the weight-loss process. By recognizing the interconnectedness of body, mind, and spirit, a more comprehensive and sustainable approach to weight management can be created.

1. Body: The physical aspect of weight loss is about adopting a balanced diet and incorporating regular exercise into the daily routine. Below are some key points to consider:

   - Mindful eating: Choose nutritious and balanced foods, including fruits, vegetables, whole grains, lean proteins, and healthy fats. Avoid highly processed foods, refined sugars, and saturated fats.

   - Exercise: Combine cardiovascular activity, such as walking, running, or cycling, with strength-training exercises. Try to devote at least 150 minutes of moderate physical activity or 75 minutes of vigorous activity each week.

   - Hydration: Drink plenty of water throughout the day to keep your body hydrated and promote metabolism.

2. Mindset: The mental aspect is about adopting a positive mindset and mindful approach to weight loss. Here are some suggestions:

   - Food awareness: Eat slowly and be aware of your body's hunger and satiety signals. Experience the pleasure of food and appreciate every bite.

   - Stress management: Stress can affect hormone balance and eating behavior. Find healthy ways to manage stress, such as meditation, deep breathing, or exercise.

   - Motivation: Identify your deep-seated reasons for wanting to lose weight and maintain motivation through realistic goals and non-food rewards.

3. Emotions: The emotional aspect concerns the investigation of emotions and behaviors related to food. Here are some guidelines:

- Emotional awareness: Learn to recognize emotions that may affect your eating behavior, such as emotional hunger or comfort eating. Look for alternative ways to satisfy your emotions, such as yoga, meditation, writing, or talking to a friend.

- Self-pity: Avoid self-pity and blame related to food. Accept that each day is a new beginning and that it is normal to have ups and downs in the weight-loss journey.

- Social support: Seek support from friends, family, or support groups that share the same weight-loss goals. Sharing experiences can help you face challenges and maintain motivation.

Incorporating these physical, mental, and emotional aspects into weight management can promote sustainable and lasting change.

10 Tips for a Healthy and Balanced Diet

1. Choose nutritious foods: Prioritize foods rich in essential nutrients, such as fruits, vegetables, whole grains, lean proteins, and healthy fats. These foods provide vitamins, minerals, and antioxidants that support your body during weight loss.

2. Control portions: Pay attention to portion sizes to avoid calorie overload. Use smaller plates, measure food quantities, and listen to your body's satiety signals to avoid overeating.

3. Balance the macronutrients: Be sure to include a combination of complex carbohydrates, protein, and healthy fats in each meal. Complex carbohydrates, such as whole grains and legumes, provide long-term energy. Lean proteins, such as lean meat, fish, eggs, or tofu, promote satiety. Healthy fats, such as avocados, nuts, or seeds, provide important nutrients and support overall health.

4. Limit added sugars: Reduce your consumption of foods and beverages high in added sugars, such as sweets, sugary drinks, and fruit juices. Added sugars can contribute to weight gain and inflammation in the body.

5. Drink plenty of water: Keep your body hydrated by drinking enough water throughout the day. Water helps eliminate toxins, regulates appetite, and promotes proper metabolism function.

6. Limit intake of highly processed foods: Avoid highly processed foods that are often high in saturated fats, refined sugars, and artificial additives. Opt for fresh, unprocessed foods as much as possible.

7. Plan meals and snacks: Plan meals and snacks in advance to avoid impulsive food choices. Create a weekly meal plan and be sure to include a variety of nutritious foods.

8. Incorporate functional foods: Add functional foods to your diet, such as chia seeds, seaweed, green tea, or turmeric. These foods are rich in antioxidants, vitamins, and minerals that promote overall health and can support weight loss.

9. Pay attention to emotional eating habits: Become aware of emotional eating habits, such as eating in response to stress, boredom, or negative emotions. Try to develop alternative strategies for dealing with these emotions, such as meditation, exercise, or writing.

10. Customize your diet: Consider consulting a nutritionist or dietitian to get a personalized eating plan. Everyone has different needs and goals, so working with a professional can help you identify the best strategies for you.

5 Tips for Stress Management

1. Practice food awareness: Develop mindfulness during meals by focusing your attention on what you are eating. Savor each bite, pay attention to feelings of hunger and fullness, and recognize your body's signals. Avoid distractions such as television or cell phones during meals and enjoy the present moment.

2. Meditation: Spend time on daily meditation to reduce stress and foster greater awareness. Meditation can help you develop a more balanced relationship with food and manage food-related emotions. You can start with short meditation sessions, focusing on breathing and letting go of thoughts.

3. Breathing techniques: Learn different breathing techniques such as deep breathing, diaphragmatic breathing, or controlled breathing. These techniques can help you relax, reduce anxiety, and stabilize emotions. You can apply them during times of stress or before meals to encourage greater awareness.

4. Practice self-compassion: Cultivate an attitude of kindness and compassion toward yourself. Accept your body and your imperfections without judgment. Be aware of your thoughts and replace negative ones with positive affirmations. Practice self-care by making time for yourself and for activities that bring you joy and satisfaction.

5. Create a self-care routine: Set aside time each day to take care of yourself. This can include activities such as a relaxing bath, a walk in the fresh air, reading a book, practicing gratitude, or any other activity that helps you rejuvenate and cultivate overall well-being.

Remember that each individual is unique and it can be helpful to experiment with different techniques to find the ones that work best for you.

INTEGRATION OF CHAIR YOGA INTO DAILY LIFE

Practical Suggestions

Chair yoga can be easily integrated into your daily life, even when you are busy with work, travel, or just want a moment of relaxation. Here are some tips to help you incorporate chair yoga exercise into your routine:

1. Workplace breaks:

   - Take a 5–10-minute break every hour to perform some simple chair yoga poses. You can do some twists, stretch your back, lift your legs, or do some deep breathing.
   - Use your break time to practice mindfulness. Sit comfortably in your chair, close your eyes, and focus your attention on your breathing. Relax and let go of the stress accumulated during the workday.
   - Use a stable, sturdy chair as support to perform some yoga poses during coffee breaks or downtime. You can do forward bends, side bends, or back rotations.
   - Do shoulder and neck stretching exercises to relax tight muscles after long sessions at the computer. You can perform shoulder rotations, arm lifts, and neck stretches.

2. Travel:

   - If you are traveling by plane, use the flight time to perform some chair yoga positions. You can do some forward bends, stretch your arms and legs, or perform some ankle rotations.
   - During a car break en route, find a safe area to park and take advantage of the vehicle's chair to do some simple yoga poses. For example, you can do twists or leg lifts to promote circulation.

3. Moments of relaxation:

   - Practice mindful breathing by sitting comfortably in a chair. Breathe deeply, filling your chest and abdomen with air, and then slowly exhale. Focus on the rhythm of the breath to relax the mind and body.

- Take advantage of relaxing moments at home to create a short chair yoga session. Light a scented candle, create a peaceful atmosphere, and set aside a few minutes for yourself to practice some postures that promote relaxation and well-being.

4. Involve colleagues:

- Organize chair yoga sessions with your colleagues during your lunch break or after work. Choose a common area, such as an empty meeting room, and invite your colleagues to participate in a short chair yoga session. This way, you can share the benefits of exercise and promote an environment of well-being in the workplace.

Remember, the important thing is to find ways to adapt chair yoga to your daily life in a practical and accessible way. Experiment with different postures and find what works best for you. The goal is to create moments of mindfulness, relaxation, and movement that contribute to your overall well-being.

10 Creative Ideas for Exercising Throughout the Day

When it comes to incorporating exercise into your daily routine, it is possible to find creative ways to make the most of opportunities without spending long periods of time or using special equipment. Here are some original and practical ideas for incorporating exercise throughout the day:

1. Go up the stairs: Avoid the elevator and choose to take the stairs whenever you have the opportunity. This simple act helps activate your leg muscles and stimulates your cardiovascular system. You can also take small breaks along the way to do some stretch or toning exercises such as leg bends or heel lifts.

2. Active parking: When you drive, try to park a little farther away from your destination point so that you can walk for a few more minutes. This will give you an opportunity to increase your physical activity throughout the day. If possible, also opt to park farther away when taking public transportation.

3. Stretching moments: Take advantage of downtime during the day to do some simple stretching exercises. You can do stretches of the arms, legs, or back while standing. This helps improve flexibility and prevent muscle fatigue.

4. Active meetings: If possible, suggest conducting "walking" meetings instead of sitting around a table. Walking while discussing can be a great way to stimulate the mind and body. Alternatively, you can also take a few short breaks during meetings to do some stretching or deep breathing exercises.

5. Dance at home: Put on some engaging music and dance freely in the privacy of your home. Dance is a great way to move, burn calories, and have fun. It doesn't matter if you are an experienced dancer or a beginner, let the music carry you away and enjoy the benefits of exercise.

6. Active gardening: Spend time taking care of your garden or balcony plants. Gardening involves different physical activities such as digging, lifting, pruning, and watering plants. This allows you to exercise different muscle groups and enjoy the benefits of nature.

7. Exercises during house cleaning: Use the time spent cleaning the house to do exercises. You can do squats while moving objects, arm push-ups while scrubbing

the floor, or lunges while vacuuming. Cleaning becomes an opportunity to move and tone your muscles.

8. Outdoor activities: Take advantage of opportunities for physical activity outdoors. You can take a brisk walk during your lunch break, have a chair yoga session in a park, or organize a weekend bike ride. The outdoors and contact with nature promote physical and mental well-being.

9. Stairs at home: If you have a staircase at home, use the opportunity to do mini-exercise sessions. You can climb and descend stairs several times consecutively to work on cardio and tone your legs. Add variations such as jumping jacks, lunges, or side climbs to increase the challenge.

10. Stretching before bed: Before you go to bed, spend a few minutes doing some stretching exercises to relax your body and improve flexibility. You can do forward bends, arm and leg stretches, and deep breathing. This will help reduce muscle tension and promote a more restful sleep.

I hope these tips inspire you to find creative and fun ways to incorporate exercise into your daily life without requiring long periods of time or special equipment. Remember that every little bit counts and that the important thing is to be consistent and find pleasure in being active!

PROGRAM CUSTOMIZATION

Tailor the Program to Individual Needs

Adapt the chair yoga program to individual needs, taking into account specific health conditions or physical limitations:

1. Consult a professional: If you have specific health conditions, complex health conditions, or physical limitations, it is always advisable to consult a professional, such as a doctor, before starting a chair yoga program. They can provide you with personalized guidance and suggestions for adapting the positions to your needs.
2. Listen to your body: While practicing chair yoga, it is essential to listen to your body and respect its limits. If you experience pain or discomfort in a particular position, modify it or avoid it altogether. Each body is unique, and your needs may be different from others'.
3. Change and adjust positions: Do not hesitate to modify the positions according to your needs. For example, if you have knee problems, you can use pillows or blankets to support your joints during the kneeling positions. If you have balance problems, you can perform the positions near a wall for extra support.
4. Focus on breathing: Conscious breathing is a key element of chair yoga. If you have breathing difficulties or lung problems, you can focus on deep, slow breathing, adapting the rhythm to your ability. Deep breathing can help relax your body and mind.
5. Experiment with accessories: Accessories such as pillows, elastic bands, or blocks can be useful for adjusting positions and providing extra support. For example, you can use a pillow under your butt to lift your pelvis during hip-opening positions. Explore different options and find out which accessories work best for you.
6. Keep an open mind: Remember that your body and needs may change over time. Be flexible and adapt your chair yoga practice accordingly. Don't be afraid to experiment with new postures or approaches, always with respect for your limitations and health.

Remember, the main goal is to tailor chair yoga practice to your individual needs, promoting well-being and safety. Always follow your instincts and never force your body beyond its limits.

Monitor Progress

1. Keep a training diary: Keep a journal in which you record your chair yoga sessions. Record the length of your sessions, the positions you perform, and the physical and mental sensations during and after your practice. This will help you monitor your progress over time and identify any improvements.

2. Measure flexibility and strength: Watch your progress by measuring your flexibility and strength in specific positions. For example, you can measure the distance you can reach in leg extension positions or the time you can maintain a balance position. You can use a tape measure, a stopwatch, or simply do a visual comparison.

3. Set realistic goals: Set achievable and realistic goals for yourself. For example, you may want to improve your flexibility, increase stamina, or reduce stress. Be specific about the goals you want to achieve and establish a plan of action to reach them gradually.

4. Celebrate small progress: Recognize and celebrate small progress along the way. Every improvement, no matter how small, deserves to be noticed and appreciated. This will motivate you to continue and give you confidence in your chair yoga journey.

5. Be constant in practice: Maintain consistency in your chair yoga practice. Find a rhythm that works for you, whether it is daily, weekly, or as you are able. Even short, regular sessions can bring great benefits over time. Commit to devoting regular time to your practice.

6. Experiment with new positions and challenges: Don't be afraid to push yourself beyond your comfort zone. Experiment with new positions and challenges to stimulate your progress. You can gradually add more complex positions or extend the length of sessions. However, always remember to listen to your body and not to force it beyond its limits.

7. Seek support and inspiration: Look for communities or groups of people who practice chair yoga or have similar goals. Sharing experiences, challenges, and achievements with others can be a great source of support and inspiration. You can participate in online classes, discussion forums, or even create a practice group with friends or colleagues.

CONCLUSIONS

We have come to the conclusion of this book, but the path to weight loss and wellness through chair yoga is actually a never-ending journey. The important thing is to keep the practice consistent and to continue to devote time to yourself and your well-being. Remember that every small step you take counts and contributes to your overall progress.

We encourage you to embrace chair yoga as a healthy and sustainable lifestyle. Continue to explore new postures and sequences, and deepen your understanding of the physical, mental, and emotional aspects of yoga. Seek the support of communities of practitioners or training partners to maintain motivation and share your experiences.

Remember that weight loss and achieving wellness are not goals to be achieved quickly, but a journey of discovery and personal growth. Be kind to yourself along the way, accept your limitations, and celebrate every small success you achieve. With dedication, perseverance, and self-love, you can achieve your weight-loss goals and enjoy a healthier, more balanced life through chair yoga.

We wish you every success in your weight-loss and wellness journey with chair yoga. Keep practicing, exploring, and taking care of yourself. The power to transform your life is in your hands. Enjoy your journey!

BONUS WORKOUT

FRAME THE QRCODE AND DOWNLOAD THE
CONTENT.
YOU CAN PRINT IT OUT OR KEEP IT ON YOUR
PHONE TO CARRY WITH YOU AT ALL TIMES

GOOD TRAINING

WORKOUT PLAYLIST

THIS PLAYLIST IS PERFECT FOR MOTIVATING YOU DURING TRAINING AND GIVING YOU THE RIGHT CHARGE TO OVERCOME YOUR LIMITS

MEDITATION PLAYLIST

THIS PLAYLIST IS PERFECT FOR UNLOADING DAYS OR RELIEVING STRESS ACCUMULATED DURING THE DAY.

LISTEN, RELAX AND USE DEEP, SLOW, CONTROLLED BREATHING

Printed in Great Britain
by Amazon

31071116R00044